# Keto:

## Step by Step

By

Mazzie Wilson

*Keto: Step by Step*

Copyright © 2015 by Mazzie Wilson

**All rights reserved.**

Published by Fontneaux Publishing 2018
Eunice, Louisiana, USA



The contents of this book are not intended to be a substitute for professional medical advice, diagnosis, or treatment. Always seek the advice of your physician or other qualified health provider with any questions you may have regarding a medical condition.

# Table of Contents

# Dedication

This book is dedicated to all of the people who struggle with their weight and body image.

You are not broken. You just need the right system and a little encouragement.

I hope this book can be part of that.

# Chapter 1: Introduction to Keto

## What is the ketogenic diet?

The ketogenic diet is a way of eating that forces your body to burn fat for fuel instead of carbohydrates. In doing so, you end up in ketosis. Ketosis is the state of burning fat for fuel. Essentially what your body does is it pulls the fat from your cells, convert that fat into ketones, and then burns those ketones the place of glucose.

Ketosis is not to be confused with ketoacidosis. Ketoacidosis is a life threatening condition suffered predominantly by diabetics. It is very, very rare for a non-diabetic person to enter into a state of ketoacidosis.

Therefore, if you are diabetic, it is best that you enter into the keto way of eating or any other diet plan with the assistance and knowledge of your physician. If your physician is against the ketogenic diet and you really believe that it can help you, then it may be in your best interest to seek out another physician in your area or to try keto on your own. But if you do it independently, monitor your blood sugar and how you feel extremely closely.

The short definition of the ketogenic diet is low carbohydrate, moderate protein, and high fat.

**How low is low carbohydrate?**

You want to reduce your carbohydrate intake to fewer than 20 net grams per day. Net carbohydrates are the carbs that are left after you deduct fiber and most sugar alcohols. These are the sugars, starches, fillers, in some cases, even preservatives that you want to keep to an absolute minimum in every meal.

**Why would you want to do the ketogenic diet?**

The thing about the ketogenic diet is it can be used for so many purposes other than weight loss. While weight loss is one potential benefit of keto, it can also be used to maintain a healthy weight. It can be used to gain additional weight in the case that you are naturally underweight or you're recovering from an illness and have become underweight as a result.

Another benefit includes hormonal balance. It has been known to help women with polycystic ovarian syndrome to overcome fertility issues and regulate their cycle.

It is also known for providing increased energy and reducing inflammation in the body. Many people with chronic inflammatory conditions such as fibromyalgia or rheumatoid arthritis report that their symptoms, while they don't go away, are radically diminished when they eat this way. The lack of inflammation helps them to have less pain, less swelling, less overall difficulty.

Better sleep is another possible positive side effect of eating keto. Not only do people report sleeping better, they report needing far less sleep than before starting this way of eating.

## Why does the ketogenic diet have so many benefits?

First, we need to look at what carbohydrates do to the body and why too many are not a good thing.

When you consume carbohydrates, your body converts that into glucose. That glucose is burned for energy. However, in order to properly control the glucose in your bloodstream, your pancreas has to secrete insulin to manage it. Too many of these insulin spikes are hard on your body.

They put a big burden on your pancreas. In fact, there is a school of thought that you only get so many insulin spikes in a lifetime, and when you're eating cake or donuts or bread or pasta or potatoes frequently, you are working in your pancreas hard. In the case of diabetics whose pancreas either does not work or is impaired, it's even worse, so if you reduce the amount of glucose that your body has to work with, you also reduce the amount of insulin that your body has to produce and use in order to handle that glucose.

Another thing that happens when you eat a lot of carbohydrates is that you don't use all of the energy that they provide. Now, high performance athletes or endurance athletes may. However, it is unlikely that the average individual is going to burn all of the energy that they consume in terms of carbohydrates.

**So what happens to the excess?**

The excess is stored in your body as fat. So contrary to what we have been taught, contrary to the conditioning, especially in the United States fat does not make you fat. Fat is not the bad guy. Carbohydrates, in the form of sugars, starches and preservatives, those are what make you fat, because when you do not use all that you consume, the extra is stored as body fat.

If you do not use all the fat that you consume, it passes out of your body in the form of waste. Think about it. You eat a greasy meal. You have to visit the restroom not too long afterwards. So with the ketogenic diet, what we're doing is starving the body of external glucose. Your body will make its own. It's designed to do this.

Many of our ancestors did not consume very much in the way of carbohydrates, so it's not imperative to consume carbs if you are getting enough protein, enough fat and enough micronutrients in terms of vitamins and minerals to sustain life. By starving the body of external glucose you force your body to turn to the glucose that was stored as fat and to start pulling from those stores and using that for energy.

When this happens, your body produces what are called ketones. Those ketones are actually more efficient fuel for your body than glucose. It is shown to lead to better neurological function. People are shown to have better endurance, better strength, better muscle building, you name it, operating on ketones rather than glucose.

Most positive things are improved by the ketogenic diet. However, that doesn't mean that it's easy. So what's going to follow is a step by step guide to walk you through it starting before you have your first keto meal.

This book will walk you through to the end of your eighth week. So stick with it for two months. If at the end of two months, you don't love how you feel, you don't love how you're losing or gaining or maintaining weight, you don't love how you're eating amazing food, then feel free to change and go to a different way of eating.

But this first eight weeks I'm hoping are going to be a huge game changer for you.

Let's go!

# Chapter 2: Before You Begin

Before you get started on the Ketogenic Diet, there are a few things that you need to know and a few things you need to do.

**We will start with what you need to do.**

First, weigh yourself tomorrow morning when you get up. Go to the bathroom, strip down to your underwear, and get on the scale. This is your starting weight. This is your baseline. It will tell you where you were so that in eight weeks you can look back and see how far you've come.

Second, take pictures. Have somebody take a good headshot and a full body photo of you. Make sure you wear clothing that hugs your body shape so that you will be able to more clearly see changes down the road.

Finally, get a sewing measuring tape and measure your problem areas. Depending on where you are in your weight and fitness, and your overall body shape it could be anything from your neck to your ankles.

The areas that bother you the most are the ones to measure. For some, it's their hips and their thighs, for other people, it's their waist and their bust or their arms and their ankles. Whatever bothers you, measure.

Write down your weight, write down your measurements, keep them with your photos and put them aside. You'll be coming back to them.

**Macros**

Once you've done this, I want you to calculate your macros. Macro calculators calculate your required carbs, protein and fat intake in order to meet the calorie limit that you will set in order to change your weight. If you want to lose, you will set a calorie deficit. If you need to gain, you will set a calorie surplus.

Here are a few different macro calculators.

Take a look at them and determine which one you feel most comfortable with. They all ask for essentially the same information. They will ask for your sex, male or female, they will ask for your height, your weight, and your age.

Once you've input this information, hit calculate and the macro calculator will give you certain data. Some of this, you will adjust in order to fine tune your macros.

First, set your carbs to 20 grams. This is the magic number for ketosis within a day or two.

From there, adjust your protein macro by choosing an amount somewhere in the middle of the offered range. For instance, if it offers you 40 grams at the low end and 100 grams at the high end, you'd choose around 70 grams as your target daily protein intake.

Repeat with the fat macro.

With regard to calories, you need to decide whether to set a deficit (to lose weight) or a surplus (to gain weight). Either way, keep the percentage between 10-20%. Regardless of your deficit, keep your calories at no less than 1000 per day.

Be aware that if you are short, under 64 inches, you will need fewer calories than someone taller. So if a 20% deficit is going to put you under a thousand calories, find the deficit that puts you at or a little bit above.

**Let's talk about how macros work.**

Your macros are going to inform your food choices. To start with, you will be limiting your carbohydrate intake. In time, you will also want to meet your protein macro. However, you do not have to meet your fat macro or calories.

It's fine to stay below your fat macro because your body will compensate with the fat that you have stored. But do not go over your fat macro. Generally, if you exceed your fat macro, you're going to exceed your calories and that essentially sabotages your efforts.

The purpose of macros to inform your food choices in terms of what foods to eat and how much.

**What you need to start.**

Now, let's talk about the items that you need to acquire before you get started on this way of eating, aside from groceries.

First, if you have a smartphone, you need to download a food tracking app. These apps are used for you to stay honest about your food intake. I've listed a few different ones, however it is by far from an exhaustive list. I think new apps are coming out almost every week as this diet gains traction. Take your time, poke around on the different apps, determine which one you think you will be able to most easily stay on top of, and use diligently in order to make the best possible progress.

- MyFitnessPal

- Carb Manager

- Senza

If you are not technologically inclined, that's absolutely fine. Simply get yourself a small notebook. Preferably, buy something hardcover that's durable and that has enough pages to keep you going for at least eight weeks. So 50 pages or more and a good pen to keep with you at all times to write down what you ate, how much, and then you can look up the nutrition information.

You will also want to buy a kitchen food scale, preferably a digital one that weighs in grams. The reason you want to use grams is because serving sizes are given on nutrition labels in two ways. They are given in volume measurements like teaspoon, half cup, or quarter cup, and they are given in grams.

For instance, the label will say serving size one half cup, and then in parentheses it will say 40 grams. The nutrition label will generally also tell you whether that weight is for cooked or raw. Use that to help you with measuring and tracking your food going forward.

## Electrolytes

You'll also want to purchase is your electrolyte supplements. Electrolytes are the minerals that you need to help you mitigate the keto flu, which has to do with carb and sugar withdrawal and can make you feel really, really horrible - weak, shaky, nauseated, sleepy, and cranky.

If you manage your electrolytes well, you are not going to struggle with the keto flu. Electrolytes are sodium in the form of table salt. It does not have to be fancy salt. Standard table salt will do the trick. Potassium in the form of a salt substitute like No Salt or Nu Salt or Morton salt substitute and magnesium. The most popular is magnesium citrate, which you can get in pill, powder, or liquid form. Magnesium oxide is very easy to find and it works, but you'll need to take more because it is not as easily absorbed and used by the body.

You can get these things at your local grocery store, the food scale and the electrolyte ingredients. I will go over how to prepare your electrolytes in the next chapter.

Now you know what to do to get ready to start on this journey. In the next chapter, we'll talk about how to spend your first two weeks and a little bit about what to eat and what you need to do before week three.

# Chapter 3: Weeks One and Two

Welcome to weeks one and two. Your first two weeks will be your most challenging in this way of eating for a number of reasons. Because of this, we're going to keep it super simple by focusing on only two things, tracking your net carbs and tracking your electrolyte intake.

## Net carbs

Start with your net carbs. What are net carbs?

Net carbohydrates are the total grams of carbohydrates that remain after you subtract fiber and most sugar alcohols. Your body does not digest fiber, therefore it does not get converted into glucose. It does not get converted into body fat. So, there is no need to count it against your carbohydrate intake.

## Sugar alcohols

Sugar alcohols are different than sugar. Most of them trigger very little insulin response. This is why their carb counts aren't counted the same as sugars and starches. The body does not convert them into glucose and then store them as fat if that glucose is not used.

However, different sugar alcohols react differently with different people. For example, Maltitol, a very common sugar alcohol, is known not only to trigger a greater insulin response than most other artificial sweeteners, but it is also has a laxative effect. It can cause bloating and intestinal distress, swelling, and sometimes even weight gain.

This is why it is important to be aware of the labels on your foods so that you do not consume sugar alcohols that are going to hurt your progress.

That being said, it will take some trial and error because not all sugar alcohols affect everybody the same way. Some people can have Maltitol and have no ill effects whatsoever. Other people can not have any artificial sweeteners, including things like Stevia, Xylitol or Erithrytol without a reaction. You need to read all nutrition labels and ingredients, pay attention to your body's response and learn what does and does not work for you.

As this is the beginning of your ketogenic journey, my recommendation is that you try to avoid artificial sweeteners altogether if you can. However, if artificially sweetened treats help you to control cravings, then use them.

## Forbidden foods

The fundamental thing to keep in mind with keto is that **absolutely no food is off limits**. However, you can *only* eat the amount of a food that fits your macros. Therefore, you can only eat the amount of bread that will keep you under 20 grams of net carbs for a 24 hour period. So if your 24 hour period is midnight to midnight and one slice of bread has 12 grams net carbs, if you can have two slices of bread at noon, you can only have one more gram of net carbs for the remainder of the day.

So there are no forbidden foods. It is strictly a matter of **"does it fit your macros?"** If it does, you can eat it. There is a caveat. While you can eat those two slices of bread, understand that certain carbohydrate heavy foods can trigger intense cravings and that carbohydrates tend to trigger hunger. That is a result of the insulin insulin response they cause. Think about when you eat a carb heavy meal. You feel really full, kind of sluggish, but an hour later you're hungry again. Just ravenous, even hangry. On keto, you eliminate the intense insulin response.

This first two weeks, the main purpose is going to be to overcome your carbohydrate cravings. It's about seeing that donut at the office and not eating it. It's going to be learning to increase your electrolytes a little bit if you feel a craving coming on or eat string cheese as a snack instead of a candy bar.

As you begin tracking, be sure to weigh your food. You cannot accurately track your carbohydrate intake or any other macro unless you weigh your portions, so make sure that you pay attention to nutrition label serving sizes.

That doesn't mean you can only have one serving of a food, as long it fits your macros. You just need to go by serving sizes in order to accurately know how many carbs are in the food that you eat.

## Weigh instead of measure

The reason weighing your food is superior to using volume measurement is that the amount of food you can put into a measuring cup is not going to be consistent from one person to another or from one meal to the next.

One person might pack baby spinach into a measuring cup until there is no air between the leaves, while another person may put them in there loosely and consider that an accurate measurement.

When you use weight, it is consistent. What if your food does not have nutrition labels? Perhaps you went to the local butcher and you bought some meat and you went to the local deli and you bought cheese and that sort of thing. The USDA has a comprehensive nutrition database, and you can find the nutrition information for virtually any food. In fact, if your app shows something different from the nutrition label, the USDA database is an excellent place to double check and verify.

## Additional key points

There are a couple of key points to keep in mind toward the end of your second week.

First, note that men lose faster than women. Men and women are physiologically different and have different hormonal makeups that affect metabolism that affect weight loss and fat burning. So as you track your progress, track it against yourself only. Do not compare yourself to someone else, even if they're the same sex.

Compare yourself only to yourself. This is why you take your initial photos, measurements and weight before beginning this way of eating. As you reach the end of your second week it's time to update your progress.

On the morning of day 15, weigh and measure yourself again. Also, have a new headshot and full body photo taken. For the photo, wear the same outfit you originally wore. This will show you how much your body has changed, regardless of what the scale says.

The scale is not the end all, be all of progress. In fact, taking your measurements again will going to tell you how your body is reshaping itself. What often happens as you move past the early part of this way of eating, is that the scale doesn't move a whole lot. However, you can measure and you might have lost two or three inches.

A lot of people wonder how that's possible. You need to consider that a pound of fat and a pound of muscle do not take up the same amount of space. A pound of fat takes up the space of a gallon jug versus a pound of muscle.

Imagine a pound of fat as a gallon size jug and a pound of muscle as a 16 ounce bottle. There's a big size difference. They weigh the same, but they are not nearly the same size, so if your weight has not changed but your size has gone down, you're still burning fat. You're still losing fat. It also means that you are meeting your protein needs, that you are building some muscle.

Carrying around extra weight is a good way to build muscle. You may also be more active because of increased energy and that will also build muscle even if it's not in the form of formal exercise.

Now that you have retaken your weight and measurements, you can compare them to where you started two weeks ago. You should see a difference. A lot of people have a large loss early on. A lot of that is retained water. It's also a big motivator because you get to see that you are losing. And though your weight loss may slow down in the coming weeks, it should be steady even if it is slow.

# **Chapter 4: Weeks Three and Four**

Welcome to weeks three and four. This week we're going to add to your tracking. The reason you want to track is because it sets you up for success.

If you don't know what you're doing in terms of food intake, in terms of calorie consumption, in terms of total carbohydrates, then how can you know if you are reaching your macros? If you're seeding them?

Sure, your weight loss so far is going to tell part of the story, so will lost inches, but in order to be more consistently successful, you absolutely need to weigh food and track what you eat.

You've already been tracking your carbohydrates for two weeks. You know how to input your foods into your chosen app. You know how to weigh your foods, how to find the nutrition information. Now you just need to add one or two more bits of nutrition information to what you have already been doing.

## Tracking protein.

The first thing you want to track is going to be your protein intake. Unlike fat, protein is a macro that you want to hit every single day. Our bodies absolutely need protein. It maintains our muscle mass and it helps us to stay healthy.

In addition, you can even go over your protein macro. Online you might find a lot of scary conversations about too much protein will throw you out of ketosis because somehow magically the body is going to convert protein into carbohydrates and then convert that into glucose. It's baloney.

## Gluconeogenesis

What people are worried about is called gluconeogenesis. The thing about it is that it is a demand driven process. It is not a supply driven process.

What does that mean?

What that means is that your body will consume protein only out of need. For instance, if you're starving, not getting enough protein, then your body is going to turn to it's internal stores. Just like by starving your body of glucose, you force it to use fat for energy. Well, if you starve your body altogether, it's gonna use whatever it can find including your muscles and other structures made of protein to keep itself alive. So it does not matter how much protein you have in your system. Gluconeogenesis is demand driven. It only happens as your body needs it to happen. It is not based on consuming too much protein.

There are dangers to eating too much protein. One, it's not good for your kidneys. But if you have an odd day where you have double your macro, it's not going to hurt you. As long as you stay within your other macros, you're fine. So hit your protein macro every single day.

When you are prepping meals, when you are eating, focus on the protein part of the meal first to make sure to hit your macro, then add in the fat and whatever carbs you are consuming. So you focus on the steak first. Then the salad and the dressing.

## Tracking calories

The other thing to track is your calorie intake.

No matter what anybody says, weight loss or weight gain come down to calories in, calories out. If you take in more calories than you burn, you will gain weight. If you take in fewer calories than you burn, you will lose weight.

This is why when you calculate your macros, you use the sedentary setting.  The setting gives you the total daily calories you burn even if you never get out of bed. Using this setting  will allow you to lose weight even if you do not exercise.

Exercise will increase your calorie burn, but if you choose to start exercising while on this diet or if you choose to continue exercising while on this diet, do not count your exercise calories. Pretend you didn't exercise and operate on the food calories versus your calorie macro.

All of the information that you need, grams of protein and calories per serving, can be found on nutrition labels or on the USDA nutrition facts database. Most food tracking apps will actually calculate this information for you automatically. However, for this next two weeks, I highly recommend that you check the nutrition label or the USDA information against the app. This will help you to see how accurate your app's tracking is and you can make sure that you're getting the most bang for your buck out of your tracking. It's important to be diligent about the details if you want to be successful.

## Sources of protein

So what are sources of protein? You do not have to be a carnivore in order to get protein. You don't have to eat frankenfoods, foods that have been processed within an inch of their lives, in order to get protein.

It's not fancy, it's not magic but a primary source of protein is meat. Pork, chicken, beef, goat, turkey, whichever meat you enjoy. Meats are almost exclusively protein. Some will have fat, some may have a small carbohydrate content in large quantity. Again, nutrition facts are your friends.

Fish is another great source of protein. The exception of shellfish, shellfish tend to have more carbohydrates. They also tend to be predominantly fatty rather than protein heavy. Not to say you can't eat shellfish. Ask if it fits your macros.

Soy is a non-animal source of protien. However, a lot of people don't like to consume soy. But tofu, edamame, and black soybeans are very popular in the keto community as alternatives to, say, black beans. They are excellent sources of protein.

It has been reported in the media and elsewhere that soy has estrogen content which can negatively affect men if they consume too much.

There are two problems with this. One, they're talking primarily about processed soy - soybean oil and soy additives. The words "partially hydrogenated" are a good indication of bad soy.

Another thing that they're overlooking is the quantity that you must consume in order to suffer these issues. So if all you eat is Tofu, yes, it's something to think about. It's something to be aware of. However, if Tofu is one meal a week, two meals a week, it's not going to hurt anything or it's very unlikely to.

Of course, this is different than having a sensitivity or allergy to soy. This is for people who otherwise have no ill effects from soy consumption.

Many vegetables have some protein content. Again, the USDA nutrition facts database is your friend.

Eggs are an excellent source of protein. It does not matter if they are chicken eggs, duck eggs, guinea eggs. They're also versatile, easy to prepare, and one of the more affordable protein sources if you're on a tight budget.

Dairy products, including cheeses, have some protein. It will vary by the type of dairy and cheese.

**Protein shakes**

One final protein option is protein shakes. Make sure you check the carbohydrate content in the shakes you choose. Some have more carbs than others. There are zero carb protein powders out there. Excellent when thrown into some almond milk and maybe with a couple of strawberries or some artificial sweetener.

You can also buy different flavors so that you don't need to add anything.

We have birthday cake flavored protein powder, for instance, which I find too sweet. These shakes can help you if you're not a big meat eater. Or if you don't take in a lot of protein heavy foods, you can have a shake with lunch, or for breakfast to start your day off with almost half of your protein covered.

Definitely consider protein powders as an option to meet your protein macro.

Another reason to make protein a priority aside from hitting your macro everyday is that protein foods are calorie dense as compared to a lot of other foods.

There are 9 calories per gram of protein, so you don't want to use up all your calories and then realize you're still 15 or 20 grams short on your protein macro. So be aware that food's calorie density does have an effect on your meal planning.

What you need to do for the next two weeks is add the tracking of your calories protein intake to the tracking you are already doing. Fat will take care of itself if you're meeting your protein macro and you're staying under your carb macro and at or below your calorie limit.

Remember, if you're doing this to lose weight, you want your body to use the fat that you're already carrying in your trouble spots, so you don't need to add that to your diet unless you're finding yourself consistently hungry. For this way of eating, fat is a really great way to satisfy hunger.

Once you've reached the end of your fourth week, it is time to take your updated stats. Weigh and measure yourself. Also get a new headshot and full body photo taken.

When you do your full body photo, be sure that you wear the same clothing that you wore in your initial photo. This is going to show you exactly how much your body has changed in four short weeks, so congratulations on making it this far.

Write down these statistics. Be proud of your progress.

# Chapter 5: Cravings

For the remaining chapters, we're going to touch on specific issues that come up with regard to the ketogenic diet.

We will start with cravings.

You will experience cravings most frequently during the first two weeks of keto. It has much to do with making that transition from a carb heavy standard diet.  What can you do to handle these cravings, undo your progress and throw you off track? You have quite a few options.

## Managing Cravings

First, if you live alone or if you and your significant other or your roommate are doing this together, or if the whole family's on board, remove any and all high risk foods from your environment. Throw away the donuts and the cupcakes, lock up the the granulated sugar.

Whatever it takes, take your high carb foods - those things that you know you need to avoid - out of your environment until you have overcome your cravings. But what about "if it fits your macros?" Until you adapt to keto, it's best to avoid foods that provide little nutritional value but far too many carbohydrates.

Now, this is not always possible for people with children in the home. Even though children do fine on low carb diets since there are no essential carbohydrates, unlike essential proteins and essential fats, a lot of people don't want to force this way of eating on their children. Therefore they will still have snack foods and bread and other carbs in the house.

If that's the case for you, then sit down with your family and figure out a way to at least have those foods out of site most of the time so they're not sitting there taunting you and and tempting you.

Another way to mitigate your cravings is to stay well hydrated and keep up your electrolytes. You're going to feel better. You're going to have more energy, and by staying hydrated, it will help keep you from being hungry in as much as the food itself helps keep you from being hungry.

If you want an easy way to get your eletrolytes, use crystal light with 1/4-1/2 teaspoon of the salt and salt substitute mixture per liter. Some flavors are so sweet that the salt helps cut the sweetness and makes them taste better. In addition you get your sweet tooth satisfied so there is no temptation to cheat. However, that electrolyte option doesn't work for everyone and you have to figure out what works for you.

Another option is when you feel a craving, find a distraction. Is there something that you enjoy doing that does not involve food? Is there a TV show you want to watch? Is there an errand you need to run? Is there a book you want to read? Anything to just take yourself out of that headspace.

Take your focus off of food and put it on something else. If you can do that for 5 to 15 minutes, odds are that craving is going to go away on its own. If you're distracted or otherwise occupied, even if it's doing jumping jacks or taking a bath, then you're going to have an easier time getting through those few minutes while the craving runs its course.

The final way is not highly recommended in most cases, but it works for many people who struggle with cravings. Make a ketofied version of the thing that you're craving. There are so many websites, recipe books and other resources to help you figure out how to make favorite foods keto friendly, that there's no excuse to cave in and eat that high carb doughnut.

Believe it or not, you can make doughnuts that only have one or two grams of net carbs a piece as opposed to 25 or 30 grams of net carbs. So don't be afraid to check out recipes and experiment with keto versions of otherwise high carbohydrate foods. This can help keep you sane if you're really having a hard time with cravings.

Make keto mug muffins. Or make the mix for one and bring it with you to work. Pop it in the microwave. You have your muffin that you can eat while everyone in the office is eating doughnuts or cake. Don't feel like you have to completely abstain from foods that you normally enjoy just because their original versions do not fit your macros. Work around it and find ways to recreate those foods to fit your macros.

Cravings are likely something you're going to deal with. They will probably be worst during the first two weeks, but they're going to get easier to manage as you stick with this way of eating.

That isn't to say that they're not going to rear their head over and over throughout the process. It's just the intensity will be less as time goes by, and eventually you may find yourself looking at a standard doughnut and thinking, 'that does not look yummy to me.' That's great. That is where you want to be, but in the meantime, use these methods to deal with your cravings so that you can keep calm and keto on.

# Chapter 6: Meal Planning

Another issue that gets a lot of attention in the online keto community is meal planning.

It can seem overwhelming. People think that a keto meal has to be complicated, that it has to be extraordinary somehow because it's different from the way they are used to eating. That is so far from the truth.

When it comes to meal planning, keep it simple. Focus on your protein first. What protein are you going to have with breakfast, bacon or eggs? Both. Add in a vegetable. Are you going to have some spinach? Are you going to have some baked fish? Have it with spaghetti squash. There are a multitude of options. One popular one is to throw baby spinach into your scrambled eggs and eat it with bacon.

Meal planning doesn't have to be super complex. Nobody tells you that bacon and eggs are not just for breakfast, so eat the keto friendly food you are hungry for when you're hungry.

Some people can do what is called monomeal. That's where they eat the same thing every day for the whole week or all the time. Some of us cannot do that. We need a little bit of variety in our palates in order to stay on track and make this way of eating more enjoyable. You know which type you are. Roll with it.

Another way to deal with meal planning is to get a good cookbook. Don't shop online for a cookbook. In this case, go to a bookstore or two or ten or whatever it takes. Find the cookbook section and find the ketogenic cookbooks. Go through them, recipe by recipe, and ask yourself, is this recipe something I could see myself making or is it too complex or is it food I don't like?

When you find a recipe book that has at least at least ten or more recipes that at least look like you think you would enjoy them, that you want to try cooking, and that you can easily get ahold of the ingredients for, you've found a winner. Feel free to pick up more than one cookbook if more than one meets this criteria.

My personal favorite is Craveable Keto. Not only are the recipes relatively simple and require few uncommon ingredients, but the author also has extensive meal plans based on how people eat. She has egg free, dairy free, vegetarian and vegan menues all included using the recipes in the book. So no matter how you eat, you can get a lot out of this cookbook.

You should not have the need for a bunch of really hard to find or strange ingredients. But there are a few exceptions that tend to be common in the keto pantry. Things like heavy whipping cream, almond or coconut flour, artificial sweeteners like stevia, xylitol, and erythritol and of course electrolyte supplements.

Those are definitely a big part of the keto pantry. However, they are not absolutely reuqired. Some are harder to find than others. It's up to you what you want to do in terms of uncommon ingredients. Some people want to keep it very simple. They have meat and a cooked vegetable or meat and a salad, and that's what they eat every day. They may change up the meat, they may change up the seasonings, but they keep it extremely simple.

Other people are more experimental. They like to try new things. And so they cook various recipes that they enjoy and they try out a lot of the different unusual ingredients. They also experiment with how to make their favorite foods keto friendly by substituting ingredients.

One thing to keep in mind on this journey is that even though, on its face, the diet may seem repetitive, i.e., protein and a vegetable, protein and a vegetable, remember that repetition is not necessarily bad.

Just because you make pork twice in a week doesn't mean it's going to taste the same each time. That is why we have seasonings and spices. You can add heat and with cayenne pepper, you can add different depths of flavor with garam masala or paprika or taco seasoning. You don't have to have plain or boring food. You can make it interesting. Use lemon juice and virtually any type of spice out there. Unless you're using in quantities of a tablespoon or more per serving do not even worry about tracking the carbs in your spices.

Get creative, learn how to season food, how to make your own dry rubs and marinades that are keto friendly. Vinegar is also really great and studies are showing that it may have some carb inhibiting properties.

Meal planning on keto is not exotic. It is not complex. It's based on what you like to eat, how you like to eat it, and whether or not it fits your macros.

# Chapter 7: Emotional Eating

If you are coming from a place of being overweight and you've been overweight for all or most of your life, chances are you struggle with some eating issues.

One of the big eating issues that a lot of people struggle with, even some who don't have a weight problem, is eating for comfort. Comfort eating can be dangerous because it's very easy to go over your macros. It's very easy to lose control of how much you're consuming.

Let's address ways that you can mitigate comfort eating.

First, what is comfort eating? Comfort eating is using food to calm yourself down. Or to make yourself feel better in a stressful situation. For instance, you have some sort of tragedy in your life and you're sad, so you immediately grab the ice cream. Or you break up with your significant other and you sit there with the bag of candy and you eat the whole thing because in the moment, and only in the moment, eating that food makes you feel better.

However, you know that the next day you are not going to feel good about eating that pint of ice cream or that bag of candy and you know that it is not going to help you on your journey to better health.

So what can you do to stop comfort eating? The best thing that you can do outside of therapy is to find other activities to indulge in. Make a list of these activities during a time when you are not stressed and when you are not seeking comfort. Sit down with a notebook and a pen and think about all the things that you like to do, that make you smile or help you relax or take your mind off of your troubles. Things that are not food related.

Here are some examples:

• Watching your favorite TV shows or movies

• Exercising, even just going for a walk in nature can be very restorative

• Meditating, spending some time just clearing your mind and letting your thoughts pass by without judgment.

• A hobby like crochet or sewing or gardening or fishing.

Those are great ways to distract yourself from the urge to eat. You might want to read a book, call a friend. There are multitude of things that you can find to distract you from the desire to eat for comfort.

These are healthier coping mechanisms, healthier ways to address whatever it is in your life that is creating the stress or the grief or the anger or the fear or whatever emotion it is that you are trying so hard to deal with. Make this list, then when you feel the need to eat for comfort, pull it out, close your eyes and point at one of the itmes. Spend some time doing whatever it is that your finger lands on.

As an alternative, go through the list and the first thing that jumps out at you, you should do. If you can't do that specific activity, do something related to it. Your sewing machine is in storage? Go to the store and browse fabrics or patterns. Look up ideas for what you want to sew when you get your machine out of storage.

Want to fish, but the weather is terrible? Go check out new fishing gear or visit the aquarium. Even browse the internet for boats or read your favorite fishing magazine.

There are so many ways that you can battle this unhealthy urge. Of course, if you struggle beyond just basic comfort eating, if you find yourself bingeing, bingeing and purging, or excessively restricting your eating, then seek therapy because that moves into the realm of a serious eating disorder. Disordered eating can be dangerous not only to your physical health, but your mental health, to your relationships, even to your employment.

Find somebody in the professional realm who can help you get your eating back in order. Your weight loss can wait for a time. Your body image issues are probably part of your disorder and those will be addressed in therapy. The key thing is to remember that as much as you enjoy it, food is fuel and pleasure or comfort is not the primary purpose of eating. You're eating strictly to fuel your body, to give you the energy and the health and well being to do all of the other things in life that make life such a rich, fun, amazing, stressful experience.

Don't seek comfort in a tub of ice cream or a package string cheese or a candybar. Seek it from within yourself. Seek it from relationships with other people. Seek your comfort in living life.

# Chapter 8: Hunger

Let's talk about hunger. Hunger is what drives us to eat. Some of us are more in tune with the feel of being hungry than others. Some people interpret it as thirst. Some people interpret thirst as hunger. A unique thing happens in the ketogenic diet.

In the first couple of weeks, you may begin realizing that you simply don't feel hungry. You wake up in the morning and there's not that driving urge to stuff your face with the first thing you can find because you're so hungry. That is because your body is using fuel more efficiently. You are also filling it with foods that meet its needs, so don't be surprised to have diminished hunger in the first few weeks. It is a perfectly natural phenomenon. The only thing to do is to keep meeting your protein macro.

Meet that protein macro every single day to the best of your ability. It's okay if you're way under some days, as long as you're at or over on other days. Essentially, your weekly average should be right around your macro, so if your daily calories are one thousand and you eat 800 a day for two days, 1100 one day, 1,300 another those four days even out to about a thousand calories a day. So you're fine.

Don't necessarily use the weekly average as an ongoing tracking element, but it's a good way to ease your mind that you're not starving yourself. Don't worry about your diminished hunger. Don't force yourself to eat, eat when you're hungry, you're not hungry. Don't force it. There's no need to do so. Your body is getting what it needs. If you are trying to lose weight, you have more than adequate stores.

Have extra fat and other reserves that your body can draw from as long as you're getting your protein. And if you do that in the form of a couple of protein shakes a day for a couple of days, that's absolutely fine. As long as you're getting your protein, it's okay to just roll with your hunger and only eat when you're hungry. That being said, your hunger is going to bounce back and you're going to have periods throughout this way of eating, whether you stay with it for eight weeks or 80 years, where you're going to just want to eat all the things you're going to be rather than us. That is also normal. That is your body going through a transition during that time, watch out for cravings, mitigate them according to the guidelines that had been offered, and make sure that that is when you use fat to help you feel full.

What is meant by this? In order to use that to help you feel full, you want to do things like incorporate more fat into your cooking, maybe some sort of oil and vinegar dressing so that the oil acts as your fat. Preferably oils like avocado oil, extra virgin olive oil, grape seed oil. Those are better than your vegetable oils and your canola oil, so use healthy oil on your salad and to cook with. A lot of people are fans of putting butter on their steaks. Not Margarine. You want to avoid processed food, but actual real good butter can one pet can make a big difference between fullness and hunger.

Now, if you're a woman, a couple of things to watch out for, be advised that your cycle will affect your hunger. It probably did so prior to this way of eating anyway. I know for myself that a couple of days before my cycle I ate anything I could get my hands on and then once my cycle started for a day or two, I didn't want to eat anything. I felt like complete crap and I wasn't hungry, so be aware that your cycle will affect your appetite and will affect your fluid retention. It will affect all the things. Don't panic. It's normal. Our hormones are different than those of men. Therefore, our bodies respond differently than men's bodies.

# Chapter 9: Fasting

Now there are a couple of tactics you can consider as your hunger diminishes. One of them is called intermittent fasting.

## Intermittent Fasting

Intermittent fasting is basically choosing an eating window during the day. For instance, if you do 16 hours of fasting and eight hours of eating, you might only eat from noon to 8:00 PM. That's when you'll get all of your calories.

You'll still drink your electrolytes throughout the day because you want to keep those at the right level and you want to stay hydrated, but your food calories are all going to be between noon and 8:00 PM.

Different people choose different eating windows. Some people start with eight and 16, which is a common schedule even for people not on keto. We sleep for eight hours a night and eat during the 16 hours that we are up. Some people do 20 hours of fasting and with a four hour eating window, or 18 hours fasting and six eating. It's all a matter of what works for you.

A lot of people find it easier to do intermittent fasting on keto because then they only need two meals instead of three and they're not hungry first thing in the morning anyway, so why not?

## OMAD

Another one is called OMAD, one meal a day. This is a little more challenging and I don't recommend you do it when you're just starting out. Essentially you pack your calories and as many of your macros as possible into one big meal every day.

Maybe you eat at six every evening or between six and seven because a lot of people who do one meal a day sit down, eat until they're satisfied and then stop for 10 to 30 minutes, and then they finish their meal. So it's not necessarily that you eat only one time, but you eat one large meal in a relatively short time throughout the day and then the rest of the day is just hydration and electrolytes.

These are options because hunger is so variable in this way of eating. For the most part, you should feel satisfied but not overstuffed when you finish eating. You should also be able to go a minimum of four hours from one meal to the next without hunger, without crankiness, and without any other issues.

# Chapter 10: Exercise

A lot of people worry that they are not able to exercise on the ketogenic diet because of the lack of carbohydrates. This is absolutely false.

The ketogenic diet has actually been shown to help increase endurance and strength. So exercise while you're on keto is definitely possible.

That being said, during the first few weeks, as your body is transitioning from burning predominantly glucose to burning exclusively ketones or fat for fuel, you may find that you're not as strong and don't have as much endurance as you had prior to starting. This should only last for maybe two or three weeks as your body adapts. Don't panic.

Keep exercising, roll with it. It's going to resolve itself and then you may find that your workouts are more explosive than they ever have been.

Contrary to what you might be told, it's also not necessary to carb up prior to exercising. If you are not a professional endurance athlete, you're unlikely to be exercising to the point of needing additional carbohydrates in order to power through your workouts. All you will do by carbing up before a workout is throw yourself out of ketosis and force your body to have to start the adaption process all over again.

Another thing to consider, is that it's absolutely not necessary to add exercise to the keto way of eating in order to lose weight. You can sit on your couch every single day as long as you are staying within your macros, you will lose weight.

In fact, certain kinds of working out can cause you to stall a little bit in your weight loss journey. Don't take that as a criticism of exercise. What's actually happening instead of losing pounds is that you are rebuilding your body and reshaping your body. You're more likely to be losing inches when you exercise regularly.

Only you can decide if you want to exercise while you're on the ketogenic diet. At first you may not, but as you gain more energy and you start seeing more of the benefits of this way of eating, that can change. When it changes, don't feel like you have to jump into some heavy, hardcore bodybuilding routine or high intensity training. Do what you can. Focus on what you can do.

If all you can do is walk around the block a couple of times when you first start before you're you're winded, or you start to walk around the block a couple of times every day or every other day. Eventually you are going to improve and you'll be able to walk around the block three times and then five times and then soon you might start finding yourself jogging around the block one time and then walking the other four.

It's fine to let things progress organically. With regard to exercise, it is fine to do cardio if that's what you enjoy. It is recommended to do some weight training when you start exercising. You don't have to be power lifting. You can be using little five pound hand weights or a ten pound Kettlebell. You can do bodyweight exercises or isometric exercises to build muscle.

The reason weight training of some sort or muscle building of some sort is recommended as you move through this weight loss process is it is going to tone your body so that you end up with a shape that you like and have less loose skin. It will also be easier for you and other people to see the progress that you're making.

So exercise on the keto diet is absolutely possible, totally unnecessary, but definitely something worth thinking about. It has benefits outside of weight loss, such as increased energy, increased endurance, better health and fitness, and better cardiovascular health.

Those things are all very, very important.

# Chapter 11: All About Weight

One final thing to cover is the particulars of weight loss, weight gain and maintenance. Let's talk more about what these are and how they were achieved.

## Weight Loss

Weight loss, which has been the focus of this book, is when you weigh more than you want to or more than is healthy for you, so you take steps to bring your weight back down to a healthy weight.

Weight loss is achieved in the ketogenic diet and most other diets through calorie restriction. This starts with figuring out what your resting calorie burn is, known as your TDEEL total daily energy expenditure, which is the minimum calories you will burn even if you lay in bed all day.

Then you eat fewer calories than your TDEE on a daily basis. Even a reduction of 100 calories per day will make a difference. You are starving your body of the calories that it is accustomed to having and so it has to use what it has stored in the form of fat, to power you through your day. This is true for every way of eating that is designed for weight loss. It boils down to calories in, calories out. Nobody has found a way around the calorie.

A lot of times people think they didn't count calories and still lost weight, when what has actually happened is that they have shifted away from eating empty calories or calorie dense foods that don't provide a great deal of nutrition. Instead, they are eating more high nutrition, calorie dense foods, and in spite of not tracking, they are actually eating fewer total calories because they're giving their body more of what it needs.

Ultimately, you have to run a calorie deficit in order to lose weight. With keto, it's easier simply because you are not as hungry.

## Weight Gain

The ketogenic diet for weight gain is the opposite of weight loss.

You have your TDEE: total daily energy expenditure, and if you want to gain weight, you want to consume more calories than your body burns on an average day. That forces your body to develop more mass to store it, and if you're exercising and eating the right things, it's not going to store it exclusively as fat. You're going to build muscle mass.

There's a lot more to it. This is a simplification, but essentially you're eating an excess of calories rather than a deficit that allows your body the resources to add mass. Therefore you gain weight.

## Maintenance

This brings us to maintenance. Online, you enounter a lot of talk about maintenance if you visit different keto sites or facebook groups, though many of those tend to be very toxic, very somewhat scary environments with a lot of misinformation. But maintenance means first that you have reached your ideal weight. You are happy with what the scale says. You are happy with your measurements. You have accomplished your goal. Congratulations. Now, you want to adjust your macros to reflect this.

So if you started at a hundred and 270 pounds, but you've reached your ideal weight of 135, you want to go and recalculate your macros for 135 pounds.

Let's say you also want to increase your carbs by a small amount, say 25 grams net. You plug that in to your chosen macro calculator and then you use the maximum allowed calories, protein, and fat.

This means the tracking doesn't stop just because you've reached your goal. You can't just revert right back to the way that you used to eat. If you do, what will happen is you will quickly find that you are right back where you started.

You have changed your body, you have changed your life, you have changed your health. Don't undo it all because you miss donuts or because you miss cheesecake.

If you want to increase your net carb intake, do it slowly over the course of a few months once you reach maintenance. Start with 25 grams net carbs for the first month. Then you go up to 30. That allows you to see if it's causing any issues with gaining weight and how it's affecting other things.

Some people find that they can't tolerate high carbohydrates after having adapted to eating ketogenically, so it's up to you to figure out. It's trial and error, but increase your net carbs by no more than five gram over the course of weeks or months at a time to test the waters.

## Keto is a lifestyle

This is not something you do for a month, then go back to eating the way you used to eat. That is what got you in trouble in the first place. How you eat is a lifestyle.

Once you reach maintenance, you have the option of a bit more flexibility. You can have some days where you're above your macros and then some days where you strictly cut back and stay well below to make sure that it averages out over the course of a week.

Those changes are gonna be up to you. Those are changes that you are going to have to experiment with.

Once you reach your goal keep in mind that the ketogenic way of eating is, in fact, a long term lifestyle. The word diet makes it sound like something temporary and it's not. It's designed for you to eat good, real food every day and stay healthy, strong and at your ideal weight.

Whether you're just starting this journey and you have a long way to go, or you're nearing maintenance, it is still a lifestyle. Good luck.

If you want more ongoing information about the ketogenic diet, visit happyketowoman.com and share your stories, ask your questions and update us on your progress.

Thanks.

# Additional Information

For more information about the ketogenic way of eating, visit happyketowoman.com.

Also be on the lookout for more books from Mazzie about keto:

• *Keto Meal Planning Step by Step*

• *Keto and Fasting Step by Step*

• *Keto for Women*

• *Keto and Exercise Step by Step*

# Acknowledgements

This book was a labor of love. The ketogenic diet changed my whole life in so many ways, not the least of which is helping me get back to a healthy weight in spite of severe hypothyroid.

However, I didn't write it in a vacuum. I couldn't have done it without the help of everyone on the keto subreddit on reddit.com. That is where I learned so much about what was happening in my body and why. They also pointed me to a number of wonderful culinary and scientific resources.

Also, my husband was a great help. He took over so much of the housework and other chores while I spent time doing research, meal planning and writing. He even ate keto along with me and was able to reach his goal weight annoyingly quick.

Finally, a shout out to my transcribers, cover designer and all of the other freelancers who were integral to seeing this book into its final form.

# About the Author

Mazzie Wilson is nearing the end of her weight loss journey, using the ketogenic diet. She's excited to have moved from tired and frumpy to energetic and healthy at the tender age of 45.

When she isn't writing books or milking goats, she can be found at happyketowoman.com.

She lives on a farm in the southern US with her husband and multiple pets.